PILATES

IN A BOX

LESLEY ACKLAND

Thorsons
An Imprint of HarperCollinsPublishers
77–85 Fulham Palace Road,
Hammersmith, London W6 8JB

The Thorsons website address is:
www.thorsons.com

Published by Thorsons 2002
10 9 8 7 6 5 4 3 2 1

Text derived from 15-Minute Pilates, 10-step Pilates, and Pilates Body Power,
published by Thorsons

Editor: Lorraine Turner
Designer: Mike LeBihan
Production: Melanie Vandevelde
Photographs by Guy Hearn

A catalogue record for this book
is available from the British Library

ISBN 0 00 713383 9

Printed and bound in Hong Kong

Caution: some of the exercises in this book and the cards use chairs as support. Please use a
strong and stable chair and test to make sure it is safe before you begin.

The exercises in this book are safe when undertaken according to the instructions given. However,
the reader undertakes these exercises at his or her own risk, and the publisher accepts no liability
for loss or injury that may result, directly or indirectly, from their use.

CONTENTS

INTRODUCTION

Do you dream of a flat stomach, a longer, leaner body and superb posture? Do you wish to improve your overall appearance? If so, then *Pilates In A Box* will help you achieve all this – and more. In this book you will discover a unique bodywork system that will help you transform your body and develop a physical presence and energy that exude total confidence and grace. If you want to become healthier, stronger, leaner and more supple, my Pilates-based Body Maintenance techniques are designed to work for all ages and all levels of fitness. There is also a fully illustrated card pack showing a selection of postures from this book, including three quick exercise programmes that you can slot into a busy day.

While most people have heard of Pilates, few know exactly what it entails. Pilates is a very disciplined, focused form of exercise, designed to strengthen ligaments and joints, increase flexibility and lengthen the muscles. The main emphasis is on 'elongating' the body to create a longer, leaner and taller silhouette. However, Pilates differs from other exercise regimes by going beyond the purely physical. This is a holistic discipline that integrates the mind, body and spirit. It is a philosophy of movement that brings about mental and physical integration. My Body Maintenance system of exercises is a unique system developed from Pilates exercises.

If you have never tried this type of exercise before, you will be surprised by its apparent simplicity. The slow, controlled movements enable energy to move more freely throughout the body. The visualization techniques gently help to focus the mind so that each exercise is executed with ultimate precision. With my Pilates-based exercises there is no need for over-exertion. The emphasis is on quality, not quantity. It's not about how much you do but how you do it. This is good news indeed for those of you who have become disillusioned and bored with fitness programmes that may not suit you.

If you want to have a long, lean look, in the safest way, you merely have to follow the guidelines in this book. Most of the techniques are based on the idea of using your own body to create resistance, so there is no need for any

4

complicated props. All you need is a willing body and a curious mind. Before you attempt any of the exercises though, it is important that you first become acquainted with the underlying principles.

Body Maintenance promises no quick fixes or sudden improvements. However, with concentration and commitment, the end result will be rewarding and nothing short of enhanced physical and mental well-being.

Achieving the body you want

With Body Maintenance I believe that you can achieve the body you want in a controlled, progressive and intelligent way. Body Maintenance doesn't build bulk, but strengthens weak muscles and stretches tight ones. You can concentrate on one part of the body without straining another. Body Maintenance differs from other forms of exercise because it initially focuses on posture. Good posture is essential in realigning the body, which can have you looking and feeling taller, slimmer and well-toned.

The beauty of Body Maintenance is that it is suitable for people of all ages. Notwithstanding your level of fitness, you have the potential for achieving a supple body and reaching a level of 'wellness' that you will want to maintain. You should feel good about yourself, which involves an intelligent dialogue between your body and mind. Imagery and visualization are very appropriate tools – if you can focus on how you wish to look, the body will most assuredly cooperate. How you picture yourself is reflected in your body language which, in turn, is observed by the world at large. When that language is fluent and flowing you will be aware of it – others will comment on how well you look.

Many people do not have a positive body self-image. Women, specifically, tend to retreat from their bodies as they get older. Body Maintenance can help you achieve the body that you want, and are comfortable with, not the body someone else has judged to be acceptable. Too often we are held hostage to figures in glossy magazines, imagining them to be preferable and easily attainable. This is unrealistic, even dangerous. We should acknowledge and appreciate our bodies and work with what we are naturally given. Many people do not even consider the highly desirable aspects of themselves. In this 'media-friendly' generation we are almost brainwashed into acknowledging 'the perfect body' hype, which is merely the fashion of the moment. This can result in dissatisfaction and depression. We can transform ourselves, to reduce our self-imposed limitations and tap into our potential – using my techniques on a daily basis will stretch the mind and the body.

Very few of us are born with an anatomically perfect body. Through habitual misuse, which begins when we are quite young and continues until we feel discomfort, we can seriously damage parts of the body. Unknowingly, certain areas are accentuated and, as we get older, it is more than likely that one side of the spine will be visibly over-developed. This is when problems manifest themselves. My Pilates-based exercise programme attempts to create the best body that is possible for you, on your frame, with the understanding that there is no such thing as the perfect body. All of us have imbalances. The trouble begins when an imbalance turns into a physical problem.

For those who have repetitive strain injury (carpal tunnel syndrome), scoliosis or other problems, Body Maintenance is a superb tool to use as you begin the journey towards easing and even reversing your condition. I believe that everyone can improve, and overcome their physical liabilities, with a safe and gentle group of exercises. You will be amazed at the body's ability to respond and rejuvenate, given the correct impetus. For those of you with serious postural problems involving balance, these exercises can change not only your body, but any vulnerability you may feel and transmit to others. You will regain your confidence and not live in fear of falling or stumbling, or giving the impression of vulnerability to others who could cause you injury.

I have never met anyone I could not help with Body Maintenance. We should not tolerate a life that is limited due to 'the back', 'the leg', etc. To embrace such negative thinking is to resign oneself to a very unsatisfactory existence and lifestyle. As you begin the following exercises be patient but determined, and feel the body working towards what you have always envisioned – the elegance of a swan's neck, the supple back of a ballet dancer. Feel yourself floating, soaring as you go through your movements. Concentrate on the moment; eventually all will be remembered as you progress. Even those of you who are extremely unfit can look forward to the day you can look in the mirror and not recognize your former selves.

ABOUT CLASSIC PILATES AND BODY MAINTENANCE

The original concept of Pilates was the brainchild of a German, Joseph Hubertus Pilates. He was extremely frail and weak as a child, but was determined to regain good health. This was the start of a life-long obsession with fitness and body building, and as a young man he excelled as a diver, skier and professional gymnast. At the age of 32 he moved to England, where he made a living as a boxer, circus performer and self-defence instructor.

When the First World War broke out, his career was temporarily cut short. As a German, Pilates was interned in England for the duration of the war. He used this time, however, as an opportunity to rethink and develop his approach to fitness. The result was the first blueprint for a whole new regime, Pilates, which drew upon all the various disciplines with which he was involved. His basic philosophy concluded that the only way to achieve true fitness was through the integration of mind and body. Hence, all his techniques were based on a combination of physical and mental conditioning.

When Joseph Pilates created his unique system of exercise during the early part of the twentieth century, the lifestyle was, in many respects, healthier for the public at large. Without the profusion of cars and mass transportation, walking was not merely a preferred form of exercise but, rather, the most efficient way of getting from place to place.

Many of the injuries and disabilities of today are, in fact, caused by our very modern, machine-oriented society. Repetitive movements on computers and sitting in an office chair for the greater part of the day contradict the physiological needs of the human body. There are also, of course, factors beyond our control, such as genetic traits and unfortunate injuries, which must also be addressed. I knew that I had to expand and enhance the basic principles of Pilates.

Body Maintenance

Almost 90 years after Pilates was created, physical ailments have changed, but pain has not. Contemporary stress has induced a variety of debilitating afflictions. In 1980 I began developing Body Maintenance, a balanced system of exercise, body shaping and toning combined with mental improvement and nutrition, based on Pilates. I initially studied with Alan Herdman, who first brought Pilates to the UK. Then I began travelling regularly to New York City to study Pilates there. During my instruction abroad I became aware of a new wave of research on the human body, and I found myself looking at the way physiotherapists were working, particularly at the New York City Ballet. I had also become aware of other forms of bodywork, including Feldenkreis and the Alexander Technique.

With Pilates as the main base, I began to integrate methods from a wide variety of sources, including remedial massage, osteopathy and injury clinics, and created my own unique system of bodywork, which I call Body Maintenance. Over the last 12 years in my own studio at Pineapple Dance Studios in London's Covent Garden, I have worked successfully with people who have suffered from a variety of modern infirmities: RSI (carpal tunnel syndrome), chronic back pain (some of which stems from spinal surgery), HIV-related problems, aerobic sprains, extreme obesity, even low self-esteem.

Often called 'yoga with machines', the Pilates-based exercises in my studio can incorporate balls, ropes, springs and pulleys. However, the most important and long-lasting work takes place on the floor. Mat exercises, essential to body mobility and endurance, target weak, under-utilized muscles in the abdomen, lower back, arms and legs. Based on mat work, the exercises in this book and in the card pack are straightforward, concentrated movements that don't need a gym or special equipment. What they do require are a few minutes – in the morning, during lunch, or later in the evening. This is a complete exercise regime devised for individuals who might not have the inclination or opportunity to seek out my studio, but who want to benefit from my tried and proven Pilates-based Body Maintenance programme.

For those of you who wish to enhance or change some aspect of your bodies, this routine is simple and straightforward. People tend to use their big muscles for everything. I work on strengthening the smaller muscles, which can give you the shape that you want. You can tone your stomach, thighs and arms and reshape your buttocks as well. Get into swimsuit shape – look and feel longer, leaner and more glamorous. There is no limit to what you can expect to achieve. My workout will have you feeling supple, slender and self-assured. Your entire view of yourself, both physically and emotionally, will improve and you will reach that summit of 'wellness' where the mind-body-spirit positively connect. The rest is up to you.

BRIDGING THE GAP BETWEEN MIND AND BODY

The main principle of Body Maintenance is that exercise is essentially a mind-body technique. Therefore, when you exercise you should mentally focus on the muscle groups that you are using. Body Maintenance recognizes that it is only through the synchronizing of thought and action that an exercise is truly effective. In order to create a healthy and fit body you need to integrate the mental, physical and spiritual spheres.

Mind over matter

It has long been established that the mind has an enormous influence on the health of the body. Research shows that the mind has an infinite capacity to induce positive physiological effects, which have both an internal and external effect. You may have noticed that when you're in a good mood you automatically seem to look and feel better. Scientists ascribe this phenomenon to the activity of the billions of nerve cells in our brain, which transmit chemical messages to the rest of the body. Our thoughts and emotions play a vital role in influencing this intercellular communication.

Think for a moment how you feel when you are stressed. Not very pleasant. This is because your body produces an excess of 'stress' chemicals (for example adrenaline and cortisol) which causes your whole system to speed up. Your heart beats faster, your blood pressure goes up, your breathing becomes rapid and shallow. At times, this type of response is necessary. It is what motivates you when you are faced with a crisis. In large doses this type of reaction can, however, be extremely harmful and lead to all sorts of unpleasant symptoms such as dizziness, shaking, profuse sweating, insomnia and migraines. It is easy to see what effect negative, stress-inducing emotions can have.

Positive feelings of calm and contentment have a much more beneficial effect, as they induce the body to produce health-enhancing, feel-good chemicals (for example endorphins and serotonin), which are vital for well-being. They promote a sense of serenity – you breathe more easily and deeply, your heart rate is slower and your blood pressure lowers. The more relaxed you feel, the less tension you hold in the muscles throughout your body. This has a beneficial effect on your general bearing and posture. Tight, tense muscles make your body shrink and constrict. This stops the energy from flowing freely throughout the body and, in time, this will be reflected in a weak, misshapen musculature.

Mindful exercise

If thoughts are so powerful, it makes sense to harness your thinking to bring about positive changes in your body. This is the essence of Body Maintenance. By learning to execute each exercise correctly you are also allowing your mind to exert a greater influence over your body. With Body Maintenance you only do a limited number of repetitions. You do them slowly, to concentrate more clearly on directing your energy towards what it is that you are trying to achieve. If you view your body in a negative way you will need to reverse your direction of thought. Positive thoughts bring about positive changes.

To ensure that an exercise is of real benefit and will bring about the changes you desire – for example a strong, straight back – you need to complement each physical action with a mental focus. By practising creative visualization regularly, you will gradually develop the intellectual and emotional ability to internalize the physical changes you wish to make. Once you've done this, the external changes will start to appear.

As you become aware of your body and its needs, you can consciously start to make changes through exercise. Body Maintenance is based on lengthening and stretching the body to its full potential. This eventually creates a longer, leaner shape, increased flexibility and a suppleness that promotes a greater ease of movement. These exercises concentrate on strengthening weak muscles and stretching those that are too tight and constricted. What you really want is a body in which strength and flexibility complement each other. It is possible to totally restructure the way you are. It is not, however, just a matter of getting your body to make the right moves. An integral part of Body Maintenance is the way you perceive the exercise. This is why attitude and creative imagery are so important. Each time you work through a series of movements, it is essential that you can envision what it is that you wish to achieve. Painting a picture in your mind helps your body to respond in the right way. This makes the whole process more stimulating and makes the effect of each exercise much more powerful. Initially it may take a while to fully understand the mechanisms. I always tell a new client to expect to do only about 30 per cent of what he or she will eventually be capable of doing. It takes about 10 sessions to comprehend the technique. Body Maintenance is one of the few forms of exercise that gets progressively more difficult, but the results are worth it. In time you will look taller, slimmer and more toned.

Creative visualization

Whatever we create in our lives begins as a basic image in our minds. Many of these images are unconscious. Through creative visualization it is possible to alter these thoughts and pictures. With Body Maintenance, the idea is to create an image in your mind that will help you to focus on the area of the body that you are working. This requires a very deep level of concentration, which does become easier with practice. On a superficial level, many of the exercises appear quite simple. How you physically position your arms and legs, however, is only part of the process. Body Maintenance, unlike many other disciplines, is actually much more complex, because with each movement you must be constantly aware of what your entire body is doing. Even when you are doing movements designed to work certain muscles, such as your abdominals, you must remember to be equally focused on the rest of your body. Where are your feet? Is your body properly aligned?

Initially, this can seem quite difficult and using visualization techniques can be enormously helpful. By understanding how your body should be feeling it becomes easier to assume the correct position. Eventually, these images will arise naturally through association, without too much effort. Visualization is an excellent method to bridge the gap between mind and body. By creating mental pictures that correspond to what you are trying to do physically, you will develop a level of body awareness that is unique to Pilates-based exercises.

Basic visualization techniques

Anyone can learn to visualize. It helps if you can begin by feeling relaxed. A still mind is more conducive to conjuring up images.

1 Spend a few minutes gathering your thoughts. Try to forget about external influences such as work, what you should be doing and any worries you might have. Remember, this is your time.

2 Do some gentle stretches and focus on your breathing. Slow, deep breathing has an instantly calming effect because it helps to promote soothing alpha brainwaves. Once you are feeling sufficiently relaxed you can start your exercises.

3 As you exercise, focus on each part of your body. How does it feel? With each exercise try to perceive a specific picture. If you are trying to envision yourself on a sandy beach, focus clearly on how this feels. Do your feet feel relaxed, warm and comfortable? Are your arms hanging loosely by your sides, like a puppet? Where is your head? Think of images that will help you to get into exactly the right position.

4 Invite each image to emerge with as much intensity as possible, so that you can almost feel it. Once you have created a familiar picture, eventually all you will have to do is to focus on it and your body will automatically respond.

The aim of Body Maintenance exercises is to bring about permanent changes. You can hasten this process by using visualization techniques when you are not exercising. These will automatically help you to walk, stand and sit in the correct way.

BEFORE YOU START

The Pilates-based Body Maintenance exercises require total concentration and focus. This makes it particularly important to find a time and place to do them where you know you will not be disturbed. This might mean switching off the telephone and ridding yourself of other distractions so that you're not interrupted. You will also need to create a specific space for yourself where you can exercise. Most of us do not have the facilities to have our own private gyms! You may, however, find an area in your home that becomes your own retreat. It helps if you get into the right frame of mind. Do this by thinking – this is my time, I am creating a space within my home, within my environment, to work on my body for myself, without distractions.

When to exercise

The exercises can be done at any time of the day. You might find that you prefer to do them in the early evening, to help you unwind and loosen tight muscles after a busy day. If you find it difficult to get going in the mornings, a 15-minute session first thing may be just what you need.

Clothes

Ideally, you should wear clothing in which you can exercise comfortably, such as leggings, shorts and a T-shirt, or leotard top. Don't wear anything that will restrict your movements. Opt for natural fibres like cotton, which are cooler. You can exercise wearing socks or, if you prefer, in bare feet. If you are concerned about slipping, put on a pair of trainers. Take off any jewellery that might get in the way.

Equipment

Having picked a suitable spot in which to exercise, try to create adequate room. This may mean moving the furniture and clearing away any clutter. Before you start, check the floor for any sharp objects or stray pins. Most of the exercises require little or no equipment. It is essential, however, to work on a padded surface or a mat. This will protect your spine and prevent any bruising against a hard floor. It is probably worth investing in a proper sports mat. Alternatively, you can work on a folded, synthetic blanket. This should be about 1.5 to 1.8 metres (5 to 6 feet) long and 30 centimetres (1 foot) wide.

Some of the exercises involve using props such as a chair, sofa, tennis ball or towel. Always make sure furniture is secure. If an exercise indicates that you need a couple of light handweights and you don't have any, you can use cans of beans instead.

If possible, try exercising in front of a full-length mirror. This will enable you to check what you are doing.

Which exercises?

With the Body Maintenance Exercise Programme it is really important always to start your exercise routine with the pelvic tilts and the abdominal exercises, because you will be working from a strong centre. Even when working your arms and legs, everything is controlled from the centre. Thus, if you are standing and doing a calf stretch, you should be thinking about the location of your stomach, spine and shoulders. As well as doing some basic abdominal work, each session you do should also incorporate stretches after the relevant strengthening exercises. You can then do upper and lower body work on alternate days.

If you have a specific medical condition such as repetitive strain injury (carpal tunnel syndrome), scoliosis, sciatica or a bad back, you can benefit from doing these exercises but you should consult a qualified Pilates teacher first. He or she will be able to let you know which exercises are suitable for you and which ones you should avoid.

Sequence of exercises

1 Do all the pelvic tilt and abdominal exercises at the beginning.
2 Proceed to the back exercises.
3 Do leg exercises and stretches.
4 Finish with upper body exercises and stretches.

Read all the instructions carefully. Remember the breathing instructions. Continue to add exercises each day as you feel more comfortable. Use your own judgement. If you are unsure, do the pelvic tilts and abdominal exercises, then add to them. If you feel any discomfort in your back during any particular exercise, you still have insufficient core strength to do it.

In Body Maintenance there are a number of basic safety rules:

- Always do stretches after the relevant strengthening exercises.
- Do not attempt to do too much too soon. Increase the number of repetitions gradually.
- If you feel nauseous, fatigued or extremely breathless – stop.
- If you have any chest pains (especially when accompanied by pain in the arm, neck, shoulders and jaw) – stop exercising immediately and seek medical help.
- If exercise leaves you unnaturally tired, check with your doctor.
- The neck is a sensitive area of the body. If you cannot remember whether you have worked this area or not, it is better not to do any further repetitions.
- Always make sure that there is something you can hold onto for support when doing the balancing exercises.
- If you experience back pain – stop.
- If your muscles start shaking – stop.
- Drink plenty of fluids afterwards, especially when it is hot.

Before you embark on any new programme, it's a good idea to consult your doctor. A pre-exercise check-up is strongly advised if you are over 40 or have not been exercising regularly. Always seek the advice of a specialist if you have a medical condition, are pregnant or have any chronic joint problems.

ESSENTIALS

Pilates-based Body Maintenance is a very precise system of exercise. It is different from other regimes in that it requires a bit of groundwork before you start. In order to understand fully what you are doing it is important that you first become acquainted with the basic principles. There are six essential guidelines to remember.

Breathing

In dance a lot of emphasis is placed on the relationship between breath and movement. However, the importance of breath is rarely addressed in the gym. Body Maintenance differs from conventional forms of exercise in that it concentrates on the correct use of breathing for each and every exercise.

Breath nourishes the body and the brain. People tend to breathe shallowly into their upper bodies when they inhale, into the upper chest and not right down into their lower lobes. If you are breathing deeply, you're working from the inside out. You are energizing and replenishing large areas of your body. Again, it is as much a spiritual as a physical idea.

For most of the exercises in this book, you will breathe out on the point of effort. During the exercises think about oxygen as a rejuvenating life-force. If you have a tight area, try to breathe into that – breath is another form of liberation, working from the inside out. Most people are stronger on one side than on the other, looser on one side and tighter on the other. You are using exercise and breath to create equilibrium in the body.

Control

All the exercises in Body Maintenance are controlled. In this particular instance the word 'controlled' means that the correct body parts are being used. Many people who think that they are using their abdominals during an exercise are in fact using their bones or hip flexors. Thus, the muscles that should be targeted are not being worked in an efficient way.

Control and precision go together. All these exercises are done slowly, in a meditative fashion. You focus the mind on what you're doing, and don't allow it to wander. You use breath, coordination, control and precision to do a limited number of repetitions well.

You minimize the stress and involvement of other parts of the body. It's preferable to do even five repetitions in a slow and regulated way, than to go through hundreds of motions, during which time nothing effective has happened. In the pelvic tilts, you should be able to feel, literally, one vertebra at a time. The fact that you do 10 repetitions in Body Maintenance well is better than doing many repetitions badly.

The same principle applies when you are using free-standing weights. In this case, you should be thinking about using internal resistance rather than using your shoulders or snapping your elbows as you use the weights. Focus on the muscles you're using, while making sure that the rest of the body is relaxed and aligned. People often make what is a simple exercise into something quite tortuous, thus creating distortion, tension and the inability to minimize the movements of other parts of their bodies.

Centring

In many Eastern religions, the centre of the body is not the heart, but the pelvis. The main principle of the Body Maintenance technique is to recognize that there is one strong, core area that controls the rest of the body. This is located in that part of your body that forms a continuous band at the back and front, between the bottom of your rib-cage and across the line of your hip-bones. This is called 'the centre'. This is the area in which the muscles in your stomach and back are – at the centre of your body. These muscles support the internal organs and keep you upright. If you have a strong centre you have a strong back, which means you can walk, stand and run without discomfort or pain. Your arms and legs are extensions of this part of your body. If you have a bad back this is an indication that the centre is not strong enough. Originally human beings were not designed to stand upright. The only reason we stand at all is due to these specific muscles. We are constantly fighting gravity, which pulls us forward. This explains why so many people have all sorts of problems with those muscles affiliated with the shoulders and neck. We are basically defying nature, gravity and our initial body type.

Flow

Each movement in Body Maintenance is designed to be performed in a smooth, flowing, undulating way. There is no room within this regime for any sharp, jarring movements or quick, jerky actions – these are the total antithesis of everything you are trying to achieve. If a movement ever feels like this, you can be sure that you are doing it wrong. Every motion originates from a strong centre and flows in a slow, gentle, controlled fashion, thus warming the muscles and causing them to lengthen and open up the spaces between each vertebra in the spine so that the body expands to create a longer, leaner shape.

Precision

In order to be effective, all Pilates-based exercises have to be performed with exact precision. This attention to detail is important because it ensures that each movement is working the body in the correct manner. Before you start an exercise sequence, read the instructions carefully. Pay full attention to proper alignment and check what the 'watchpoints' have to say. This will ensure that you do not expend excess energy doing an exercise incorrectly.

Coordination

Children run naturally, but for most adults basic coordination is a major problem. Many people, when starting Body Maintenance complain to me, 'I can't coordinate my breath and the movement. It's too much. I've got to concentrate too hard. I can't do it.' Most of us have lost the ability to coordinate the mind and body into a working machine. We no longer have the sense of our feet being in contact with the earth. We've lost the feeling of the way the breath moves naturally through the body. The aim is to retrain the neuromuscular connection between the brain and the body.

This is best illustrated when I try to teach foot exercises to people. I sometimes joke that the feet are very far from the brain and they won't obey because they haven't been asked to do anything for a long time. Observe people who have lost the use of their hands. They can do the same things with their feet that others can do with their hands. We all have that capability, but we don't employ it. If you don't avail yourself of something it atrophies; if you don't use coordination in the physical sense you lose the ability.

Some of the exercises in Body Maintenance appear quite complicated; that's because they're based upon the introduction of a more complicated concept than mere physical movement. They are trying to reintroduce the mind to the mind/body equation. If I ask my opposite arm and leg to do something at the same time, coordinating from the breath and a strong centre, I should be able to achieve it. If I slip in the street, I am more likely to regain my balance than not. If someone throws a bunch of keys at me, I will probably be able to catch it. Since I have the neuromuscular connection between the mind and body parts, I can be spontaneous, and this is where the proprioceptive concept – the linking of mind and body – comes into play.

In Body Maintenance, we try to recreate your body as a coordinated whole, rather than thinking 'I am exercising an arm or leg or the stomach'. Coordination is paramount to the way the exercises flow. You might see a Body Maintenance exercise that is similar to those used in aerobic classes or at a gym, but the difference between a Body Maintenance exercise and an aerobic one is that, in Body Maintenance, the movement is concentrated exercise and requires minimal effort from other parts of the body.

Key terms

In Pilates and Body Maintenance there are certain key terms that are referred to over and over again. It helps if you understand these before you begin.

Relaxing

Pilates frequently refers to keeping an area relaxed. This isn't necessarily what you might think. Most people associate relaxation with a feeling of 'letting go', of allowing muscles to slump. In this case, to relax means to release tension in an area while still managing to maintain tone and control. This should feel comfortable and natural.

Neutral spine

Some of the positions you will be assuming require your spine to remain in neutral. This means that you maintain the natural curve in your back. Thus, when you are lying down, do not press your back so hard into the floor that you lose your natural curve. Neither must you allow your back to arch so that your lower back comes off the floor. Just lie there, breathe in and out naturally and allow your back to relax into the floor without pressing it in. This will permit your back to relax into its natural, neutral position – which is slightly different for everybody.

The centre

With Body Maintenance, every exercise originates from the centre. The stomach muscles are the core to everything and support the spine. It is important that you always remember to keep this area correctly aligned. This is particularly important when you exercise the lower abdominals because it is very easy to do the opposite of what you actually want. It is natural when you breathe in for the stomach to pull into the spine and when you breathe out for it to bulge. This is not what you want. You will have to try to reverse what the body wants to do unconsciously. As you breathe in you should relax the stomach; as you breathe out you should pull the navel to the spine, engaging the lower abdominal muscles. Your body will want to do the opposite, but it's important to engage the stomach muscles when you exhale.

The feet

The main thing to remember when exercising is that most of the time your feet should be relaxed. If you are in doubt – relax your feet. Most people tense their feet too much and as a result they constantly complain about getting cramp in their feet when they are exercising. (If you do get cramp, use a foot roller to ease away the tension.) A relaxed foot should feel comfortable, so that there is no sensation of tightness. Whenever you are required to flex your feet, do so by gently stretching out your heel then pulling the top of your foot as far as you can without straining. Do not tense your foot so that it feels strained in any way.

The neck

This is a sensitive part of the body, so you do not want to put it under unnecessary strain while you are exercising. It is very important that you always follow the neck instructions very carefully. Body Maintenance often refers to keeping your neck long, which means adjusting your head into a position that lengthens your neck. When you are doing an exercise lying on your back, the way you bring your head into alignment with the rest of your body is by moving the top of your skull and the base of your neck. Do not attempt to flatten your neck against the floor.

Straight arms and legs

This is a very common term in Body Maintenance. Your arms and legs should be relaxed and not locked. This is an important point to remember, particularly for the stretches. If an exercise requires that you stretch your arm or leg out straight, you should take care not to overextend, which causes the joints to lock.

Body basics

The main function of the skeletal system is to provide your body with support, protection and movement. Bones act as levers and when muscles pull on the bones, this causes parts of the body to move. Muscles are attached to the bones by tendons composed of tough, fibrous, non-elastic connective tissue. The bones you should be most concerned about in Body Maintenance are the main 28 bones that comprise the spinal column, consisting of:

- Seven cervical vertebrae in the neck.
- Twelve thoracic vertebrae articulating with the ribs in the thorax.
- Five lumbar vertebrae in the lower back.
- Four bones that are fused together into the coccyx at the base of the spine.

One vertebra at a time

Body Maintenance frequently refers to the term 'one vertebra at a time'. This is one of the main principles that you should keep in mind whenever you are doing an exercise that involves rolling your body up from and down to the mat. The idea is that you always roll up gradually so that you are lifting only one vertebra off the mat at a time. The same rule applies when you roll back down again. This takes some practice and initially you will need to concentrate very carefully to ensure that you are doing it correctly.

Movements

All movements involving the bones occur at the joints, thus enabling a variety of different movements. The more common ones that you are likely to come across in Body Maintenance include:

- **Flexion** – which bends a limb or the spine, for example when bending the head forward onto the chest.
- **Extension** – which straightens a limb or the spine.
- **Hyperextension** – which means bending back further than the vertical position, for example moving the head backwards to look up at the ceiling.
- **Abduction** – when you make a move away from the centre of the body, for example raising your arms horizontally sideways.
- **Adduction** – when you move towards the centre of the body, for example you lower your arms to the sides.
- **Inversion** – when something turns inwards, for example you turn the sole of your foot inwards.
- **Rotation** – when the bone turns on its axis either away from or towards the centre of the body.

The muscles

Muscles create a movement by exerting a pull on the tendons, which move the bones at the joints. They are also responsible for maintaining posture. Many muscles are attached by the tendons to two articulating bones. Most movements, therefore, involve the use of several muscle groups. Muscles may also work in 'antagonistic' pairs – one muscle contracts to move the bone in one direction; the other muscle contracts to move it back, for example the calf and shin muscles that raise and lower the foot. Each muscle has the ability to contract or shorten. It can be stretched when it is relaxed. Muscles also control internal functions such as pumping blood round the body and the propulsion of food through the digestive system.

There are literally hundreds of muscles in the body (there are 620 muscles that can be consciously controlled alone), all of which are involved in a wide range of functions. The most important muscles you should be aware of for the purposes of Body Maintenance are:

Trapezius – in the back of the neck running down to the shoulders
Action – extends the head

Levator scapulae – at the back and sides of the neck, running into the shoulder
Action – lifts the shoulder blade and shoulder

Deltoid – on top of the shoulders and upper arms
Action – moves the arm backwards and forwards

Biceps – at the front of the arms
Action – moves the arm

Triceps – at the back of the arm
Action – moves the arm

Gluteus maximus – forms the buttocks
Action – raises the body, used in running and jumping

Gluteus minimus – in the buttocks
Action – rotates thigh laterally, maintains balance, used in walking and running

Sartorius – crosses front of thigh from lateral to medial side
Action – flexes hip and knee, for example when sitting cross-legged

Semitendinosus (hamstrings) – down posterior medial side of thigh
Action – extends thigh, flexes leg at knee

Quadriceps extensor – on the front of the thigh
Action – opposite movement to hamstrings

External oblique – extends laterally down the side of the abdomen
Action – compresses abdomen, twists trunk

Internal oblique – extends laterally down the side of the front of the abdomen
Action – compresses abdomen, twists trunk, works with the external oblique

Rectus abdominis – runs down the entire length of the front of the abdomen (divided into four sections)
Action – an important muscle for maintaining posture, draws front of pelvis upwards

Transverse abdominis – runs laterally across front of abdomen
Action – compresses abdomen

Erector spinae – found medially on the posterior surface of neck, thorax and abdomen
Action – extends the spine, holds body upright

Latissimus dorsi – runs down the back of the lower thorax and lumbar region
Action – draws shoulders downwards and backwards, adducts and rotates arm, helps pull body up

Body awareness

Before you begin the Body Maintenance programme, try this simple preliminary body awareness exercise.

Standing or sitting, close your eyes. Take a few deep breaths and, starting with your head, slowly direct your focus down through your entire body. Imagine that you are steering the flow of energy throughout your body. As you do this, try to visualize all the different parts of your body along the way. Think of your eyes, ears, mouth, down the shoulders, arms and hands. Visualize your chest, back, abdomen, hips, pelvic area, upper legs, knees, lower legs, ankles and feet. As you visit each area, try to build up a mental picture of how it looks and feels. Spend a few seconds tuning into each part. Move your head gently, shrug your shoulders. Gently move your stomach, tailbone and hips. As you do this, concentrate on the sensation. Which areas feel most comfortable and relaxed? Are certain areas tight and constricted? Do this for a few minutes each day. This will help you to become more aware of your body when you are ready to begin the exercises.

EXERCISE PROGRAMMES AND HOW TO USE THE CARDS

The exercises that follow will help you to tone and strengthen specific muscles in your arms, back, stomach, chest and legs. In time, as your body adapts, you will also start to look taller, slimmer and more youthful. The 30 cards in the card pack feature a selection of exercises that focus on the pelvis and abdominal muscles, the back, legs, and upper body. The cards also present three complete, yet quick, programmes that you can fit into a busy day. Position them wherever you can see them easily, and refer to them whenever you need to check your posture and what you are doing. Each card features clear instructions for you to follow as you perform each exercise.

Before you attempt any of the main exercises, start with the following essential posture and balance exercises. It is best to do these in bare feet. If you've got a mirror – even better. That way, if you stand sideways, you'll be able to keep an eye on what you're doing and make sure that it's correct.

PERFECT POSTURE – HOW TO LOOK INSTANTLY TALLER AND SLIMMER

Not sure if you're standing correctly? Then practise this position for a few minutes daily. After a while it will feel so natural that you no longer have to think about it.

1 Stand with your feet hip-width apart. Imagine that you're standing on sand. Your feet are relaxed.

2 Think of your weight being over the middle of each foot, with your toes gently lengthening into the sand.

3 Close your eyes and make a mental note of the following checklist:
- Don't sink back into your heels or lean forward. Keep your weight evenly distributed over your feet.
- Let your arms fall naturally in front of your body.
- Let your hands hang from the shoulders, totally loose and relaxed.
  - Don't lock your knees. They should feel relaxed and not rigid.
    - Keep your inside thighs and bottom relaxed.
      - Imagine that your head is like one of those nodding dogs in the back of a car. It's not going backwards and forwards but resting directly upon your shoulders and rocking gently until it settles into a comfortable, neutral position.
        - Think of the bones directly behind your ears. Try to imagine these bones 'reaching' towards the ceiling.
        - Pull your stomach in, without tipping the pelvis forward. Think of a piece of string from your pubic bone to your navel. It is shortening as you pull up and in. Feel your tailbone drop – as if it is weighted to the floor. This will seem much easier after you've done more of the stretches to release the pelvic girdle.
        - Keep the front of your thighs relaxed.

Now your whole body is perfectly aligned – you should feel as if you are floating an inch off the ground.

Exercises for better balance

If you're worried about slipping, tripping or not being able to catch objects thrown towards you, your sense of balance is probably poor. What seems to occur, as you get older or as a result of any injury, is that you lose your awareness of balance and your reflexes are no longer as sharp. This can cause great feelings of insecurity. Perhaps you begin to worry more about safety. We all know that the simplest of falls might have serious consequences. This is reflected in the body, which becomes stiff and constricted as a result. The easiest way to change this is to practise the following exercises every day. In time, you will start to feel lighter and more confident in the way you move.

For each of these exercises all the same rules as the Perfect Posture exercise apply (pages 27–8).

STANDING ON ONE LEG

1 With bare feet stand on both legs, and imagine you are on a beach with soft sand between your toes. Let one foot float off the ground.

2 Count for ten seconds and change legs. Repeat four times, twice on each leg.

3 Now do the same – with your eyes closed. Make sure you have something to hold on to, lest you fall over.

STANDING ON ONE LEG ON A TOWEL

Do exactly the same as in the previous Standing on One Leg exercise, this time standing on a flat towel. This gives you a slightly more unstable surface and makes the exercise more difficult. Even if you don't exercise regularly, try to do these every day – especially if you are over 45 years old.

WALKING BACKWARDS

1 Start in the Perfect Posture position (pages 27–8) and, with feet approximately 2.5 centimetres (1 inch) apart, start to walk backwards. Slowly drag your foot back, so that it never entirely leaves the floor. The easiest way to master this is to imagine that you are trying to remove some chewing gum from under your feet.

2 Look in the mirror – but do not look down at your feet. This exercise is even more effective if you imagine you are walking on sand.

Breathing

Correct breathing is a very important facet of Pilates. By remembering to breathe properly, you'll find it becomes much easier to exercise. The problem is that most people don't breathe deeply enough. Breathing slowly and deeply is very energizing. It ensures there is sufficient oxygen circulating throughout the body.

It may sound obvious, but when you exercise do not hold your breath. It's better to breathe incorrectly than not at all. Practise the following exercise before you start any of the stomach work.

BASIC BREATHING EXERCISE

1 Lie on your back in a relaxed position, resting your head on a folded towel, with your knees bent.

2 Place one hand on your stomach and, very gently, breathe in through your nose. Feel your lungs filling with oxygen and slowly expand and relax your stomach. Breathe out.

3 With one finger on your pubic bone and one on your navel, try to shorten that gap as you breathe out, and flatten your stomach to your spine without tilting your pelvis.

4 Breathe in again and feel that gap slightly expand.

5 Breathe out. Imagine there is a piece of string or an elastic band that links your pubic bone to your navel. Very gently feel it pulling up and in. This will get all three sets of stomach muscles working, including your oblique muscles, which will tighten your waist.

Make sure you breathe slowly and deeply. One of the main rules of Pilates is to breathe out on the point of effort. If in doubt, particularly on the stretches – breathe naturally.

When you breathe in your stomach gently expands. However, it shouldn't swell in an exaggerated way. Try to think of your ribcage expanding gently to the sides so that you're not just breathing into your throat and upper chest.

When you begin this exercise programme and you start to breathe properly, you might find that you feel a bit dizzy. As you are learning to breathe more deeply, you are taking in more oxygen, which can make you feel light-headed.

ABDOMINAL AND BACK EXERCISES

Women are often obsessed with having flat stomachs like men, regardless of the obvious physical differences. These exercises, combined with careful and healthy eating, will tone and tighten the stomach area. They will not make you lose weight, but they will give you a flatter, leaner stomach.

As people age, their metabolism changes and they must exercise more to burn up the same amount of calories. By exercise, I mean walking instead of taking the car or a bus, or climbing the stairs instead of taking a lift. If you're short-waisted and eat large meals, you are going to have a stomach that protrudes. It is better for your blood sugar levels to eat small amounts throughout the day. Also allow yourself some flexibility, and don't obsessively deny yourself certain foods.

In Pilates when you do your abdominal work, as you breathe in the stomach gently expands. As you breathe out the stomach pulls in, navel to spine. Feel the connection from the pubic bone up to the navel. The body will automatically want to do the opposite as you breathe out. You inhale through the nose and exhale through the mouth. As you breathe out think about pulling the navel to the spine without tipping the pelvis. If you have trouble with the pelvis and you have tight hip flexors and glutes, go to the section of the leg stretches where you stretch your bottom with the foot on the thigh (pages 60–2), and do one or two of those stretches first to relax your pelvis.

A strong stomach exists to support your internal organs and back. The taller you stand, the more balanced your stance, the flatter your stomach will appear. When you are posturally aligned and maintaining an erect back while walking, you are exercising your body perfectly well. If you sit slouched all the time and if you walk with a slump, your stomach will stick out. These abdominal and back exercises are good for conditioning, toning and strengthening. They're also good for anyone with a bad back, sciatica or scoliosis. If you have any of these problems you need to do abdominal and back work, but do not attempt any of the advanced exercises at first.

It's better to do these exercises either lying on a towel or on an exercise mat. As you're lying on your back, you may want to place a folded towel under your head. This will help lengthen your neck. If you're not sure about this, try it with and without a small folded towel and see which is more comfortable.

Repeat each exercise 10 times. Do the stretches in sets of four. Stomach muscles have an unusually short memory. Daily reminders will keep them taut and toned.

PELVIC TILT

The pelvic tilt is a preparation exercise that warms up the back. It's a good starting point, whatever part of the programme you plan to do.

1 Lie on your back, with your knees bent and parallel, about hip-width apart. Arms should be resting at your sides, with palms facing the floor. This helps to lengthen your neck.

2 Breathe in, then breathe out and gently relax your back into the floor. When you do this, do not press your back too strongly to the ground so that you lose your natural curve. Do not allow your back to arch to the point that it lifts off the floor. This is called the neutral spine position and it is slightly different for everybody (page 21). There is no point in trying to force your back down. Try very hard not to tense your buttock muscles during this exercise.

3 As you breathe out, gently tilt your pelvis forward and roll your lower back off the floor – one vertebra at a time, as you 'peel' your back off the mat (page 23).

4 Breathe in, keeping your neck long, and very slowly roll all the way down, breathing out. Keep your feet relaxed on the floor and imagine that your toes are 'lengthening' away.

PREPARATION FOR ABDOMINALS

This is a preparation for the abdominal exercises. It will wake up your stomach muscles and prepare you for the more difficult exercises.

1 Lie as before in the Pelvic Tilt exercise (page 34) – with a relaxed back and long neck, without tucking the pelvis under. Take either a small cushion or folded towel and place it between your thighs. Very gently breathe in through your nose.

2 As you breathe out, feel your stomach muscles pulling down to the floor. Think of them pulling up and into your spine. Hold your breath and count to four. Squeeze the towel or cushion with your thighs. You can put your fingers on your stomach if you wish so that you will be able to feel the muscles you are working.

3 As you breathe in through your nose, feel your stomach gently expand into your fingers.

4 As you breathe out, feel your stomach pull away from your fingers. Feel your lower abdominal muscles working. Think of working on the transverse and the rectus abdominis muscles first, and the obliques second. Repeat 10 times.

Watchpoints
• Don't let your pelvis lift off the floor. This will 'shorten' the neck. Watch that your stomach doesn't 'bloat'. Instead, make sure that on the point of relaxation – when you breathe in – the stomach gently lifts. As you breathe out you should feel your stomach pull up and in, away from the pubic bone.

• Most people naturally want to breathe in and pull their stomach muscles in – this is a mistake. As you breathe in, you gently soften the muscles as they flow out into your fingers. As you breathe out, the stomach pulls away from the fingers. Think of it as pulling 'up and in'. This will help you focus on your lower abdominals – strengthening and toning that area.

WORKING THE LOWER ABDOMINAL MUSCLES

1 Lie in the same position as in the Pelvic Tilt exercise (page 34), with your knees bent. Place your hands on your hip-bones. This helps to stabilize your pelvis.

2 Begin with the right leg. Keep your left leg completely still. Very gently breathe in and let your right knee open sideways. As you breathe out feel the resistance. Bring the leg back to the other one – breathing out and pulling your stomach in.

3 Change legs. Now, breathing in, open the left leg to the side. Exhale and slowly close. Repeat 10 times, alternating legs each time.

Watchpoints
• Think of the muscles between your navel and your pubic bone as a fan. As you inhale and the knee opens, the fan opens. As you exhale, the muscles tighten and the fan closes.
• Do not tilt the pelvis, and make sure that the supporting side is stable.
• Do not press your back into the mat.

WORKING THE LOWER ABDOMINAL MUSCLES 2

This slightly harder version of the previous exercise is very straightforward.

1 Interlace your hands behind your head (this will help prevent you from straining the muscles in your neck). Slide them high up behind your skull. Do not let them slip to the neck. Keep thumbs on either side of your spine.

2 Lift your elbows so that you can just see them out of the corner of your eye without moving your head. When you can see your elbows peripherally you know that your arms are in the right place.

3 Very gently exhale and 'float' your head and shoulders off the mat.

4 Hold that position and repeat the previous exercise. Repeat the exercise 10 times, five times on each side.

Watchpoint
• As you lift your head, your focus shouldn't change, so you don't shorten your neck. If you shorten your neck you may tip your pelvis. This will make it very hard to work your lower abdominal muscles. You may also place a strain on your lower back and your body will be incorrectly aligned.

BASIC ABDOMINAL CURL

This exercise uses exactly the same position as the previous exercise, although the knee does not fan out. All the same rules apply.

1 Lift your elbows up where you can see them in peripheral vision.

2 Keep looking at the ceiling and gently breathe in through your nose. Relax the abdomen, but do not 'bloat' it out.

3 As you breathe out, gently lift your head and shoulders off the mat. Only go as high as you can. Do not strain your neck in order to hold that position.

4 Breathe in as you go back down again.

Watchpoint
• As you breathe out, try to imagine that a piece of string is pulling you up from your pubic bone and under your rib cage. Pause until all three sets of abdominal muscles go 'up and in', and flatten.

SINGLE LEG STRETCH

This stomach exercise is a simple single leg stretch. It is the first really coordinated exercise. It is a simple and basic exercise – which is not the same as saying it is easy.

1 Lie on your back, with your knees bent and parallel, about hip-width apart. Interlace your hands behind your head. Lift your head and shoulders gently off the mat.

2 As you breathe out, slide your right leg down, approximately six inches off the floor.

3 Breathe in, putting your head and shoulders down and bringing your right leg back up.

4 Breathe out, lift your head and shoulders, and slide your left leg down, approximately six inches off the floor. Repeat 10 times, alternating the legs.

Watchpoints
• Many people make the mistake of exhaling before curling forward. If you do this, you will not get the same benefit. You exhale as you do the exercise.
• Remember to keep looking at that same point on the ceiling. If you pull your chin into your chest you may strain your neck and won't get the results you want.

BASIC SIT-UP

1 Lie on your back with your legs comfortably against a wall or with your feet held up by a friend. Be close enough to, or far away enough from, the wall so that your tailbone is weighted to the mat. If your bottom is off the ground you're too close to the wall. Conversely, if you're too far away your legs won't feel supported.

2 Take your hands behind your head and lift your elbows to where you can see them in your peripheral vision. Keep the neck long.

3 Very gently breathe in to prepare. As you breathe out, lift the head and shoulders off the mat, pulling your stomach towards your spine.

4 Pause, breathe in and lower. As you breathe out and lift, the stomach pulls in, the pelvis does not lift. The neck is long, the head is cradled in the hands. You are not pulling your chin to your chest. Think of the breast bone and the head as floating off the mat. Don't think of a sharp pulling movement.

Do 10 repetitions.

Watchpoint
• Hands are interlaced high up behind the cranium and are not placed behind the neck.

ADVANCED SINGLE LEG STRETCH

This is the most difficult exercise in the programme, because it is an exercise with both legs off the ground. If you have any back injuries at all, don't do it until you feel strong enough.

1 Lie on your back, with your knees bent and parallel, about hip-width apart. Interlace your hands behind your head.

2 Bend both knees into the chest and allow your tailbone to be relaxed and heavy. Look at the ceiling and breathe out. Let your head and shoulders 'float' off the ground, depending on how much mobility you have. Inhale.

3 Exhale and stretch one leg out, pulling your stomach into the spine.

4 Inhale and bring the leg back.

5 Exhale and extend the other leg.

Do five stretches on each leg. If you wish you may relax at the end and do another set. Only take the leg as low as the point where your back does not arch away from the floor. The lower the leg, the harder the exercise.

SIDE STRETCHES, SIDE LIFTS AND BACK EXERCISES

The first three exercises in this section are also for the abdomen but they are done lying on your side. These are called side stretches and side lifts. They are particularly good for the waist obliques. The same rules apply as for all the abdominal exercises. It doesn't matter which side you lie on to start with. Do all the exercises in sets of ten. Those that follow are for the back.

You cannot stand upright if you have a tight, weak back. Any minor adjustments that you make to try to correct the way in which you walk, sit and stand will only create further problems. Gentle exercise and control are the key. If you envision these exercises as stomach exercises, you can't go wrong. If you think of them as back exercises, however, the result will be frenetic movement that won't accomplish much except possibly 'concertinaing' your bones.

If time allows, the lower back exercises should be done after the stomach exercises. These exercises work better as a pair. You must strengthen your stomach before you start working on your back, because the abdominal muscles initiate the work needed to develop a strong back. All exercises are directed from the abdominals.

SIDE STRETCH

1 Lie on your side, arm stretched out in line with your body, resting on the floor, palm down. Place your other hand on the floor in front of you, for balance. If your neck doesn't feel comfortable, place a folded towel between your ear and your shoulder.

2 Think of your ear 'lengthening' along the arm, so that you're looking directly ahead of you. The hips are stacked one directly over the other so that your pelvis is level, not tilted. It's very common to let the top hip rock forward. Glance down your body without moving your head. If you can't see your feet, they are too far behind you. If you feel any strain in your back, the first thing you should do is move your feet further forward.

3 Breathe in to prepare. Breathe out and lift your legs about 10 centimetres (4 inches) off the ground. Keep your feet gently flexed. Straighten the back of your legs. Feel the energy pushing through your heels as you lift. Breathe in as you lower. Do 10 on each side.

Watchpoints
• If you are unsure about this position, do it with your back against the wall. You can then feel how far your legs have to come forward to feel your middle back against the wall.
• Stretch your legs as far as you can without locking your knees. The knees are lengthened away, but slightly relaxed. If you're not sure about locking your knees or stretching your knees, it is always better to have them slightly released.

SIDE STRETCH 2

This exercise is simply a harder version of the one before – so all the same rules apply. Use a towel if necessary.

1 Relax your top arm and shoulder. With flexed feet, breathe out and think of your legs floating off the ground. Hold this position and breathe in.

2 Breathe out and lift the top leg.

3 Bring the leg back, breathe in, and slowly lower both legs to the ground and relax.

Do 10 repetitions on each side.

Watchpoints
- It's really important for this exercise that you never allow one leg to become longer than the other. You don't want an imbalance in your pelvis.
- Correct breathing is vital. If you feel any strain in your back, try doing the exercise with your legs further forward.

SIDE LIFT

This exercise is more difficult and you need to be reasonably fit to try it. Don't attempt it if you have any back injuries.

1 Lie on your side, with your elbow directly under your shoulder, and your palm flat on the floor. Keep your legs in a straight line with your ankles crossed. It helps if you can place your feet against a hard surface – for example a skirting board, or the bottom of a sofa. This will give you a bit of resistance and help you get off the ground. All the same rules on alignment apply as in the side stretch. Keep your shoulder and elbow in line.

2 As you breathe out, lift, pushing down through the supporting arm. The other arm lifts up to a right angle in line with the shoulder.

3 Come back down and relax.

Begin by doing this exercise four times on each side and slowly build up to ten. This will give you a strong, toned and, hopefully, very trim waist.

Watchpoint
• Don't allow the top arm to swing behind you. This is a common fault, and can cause the body to rock backwards.

CAT STRETCH

A cat stretch is done on your hands and knees.

1 Make a square of your body. Keep your hands under your shoulders, fingers facing forwards with your hands shoulder-width apart. Knees should be hip-width apart. If your knees feel a bit uncomfortable, just fold up a towel and put it under them. Place your feet gently on the floor and don't lock your elbows at any point.

2 As you breathe out, drop your chin to your chest and curl your stomach into the spine. Press your upper back to the ceiling, trying not to rock back and forth.

3 As you breathe in, your tailbone lifts towards the ceiling, your chest presses to the floor and your head gently lifts.

4 Breathe out and reverse the position.

5 After 10 repetitions, relax your bottom onto your heels and just breathe. This is called the 'relaxation position'. You can do this relaxation at the end of the sequence of back exercises, or at the end of each back exercise.

Watchpoints
- Don't lock your elbows.
- Don't lift your head too high or you may strain your neck.
- As you press your chest down to the floor (in the reverse exercise), if you feel any pinching in your lower back you'll know you've gone too far.

BACK STRENGTHENING

1 Lie on your stomach with your feet relaxed. Your arms should be facing forwards and be just wider than your shoulders, which are relaxed. Keep your neck 'long' by looking down.

2 Keep looking down as you gently press your hips into the floor and pull your stomach in.

3 Gently, lift your head up (keep it independent of the body), focusing your eyes on the same point. Keep your feet on the floor.

4 Breathe in, and gently come down. Feel your buttocks contract slightly. Do not contract them too much – otherwise you're using your buttock muscles and not the stomach. Engaging the abdominals helps to strengthen your back and lift your body.

5 As you breathe out and lift, imagine that the crown of your head is going forward towards the wall in front of you. Do not lift your head towards the ceiling. Ideally, you want as little pressure on the hands as possible.

6 Relax your fingers and feel your shoulder blades releasing. Relax down again.

BACK STRENGTHENING 2

This exercise is exactly the same as the previous back strengthening exercise (page 47), except that this time, as you breathe out and lift, your hands 'float' off the ground.

1 Lie on your stomach with your feet relaxed. Your arms should be facing forwards and be just wider than your shoulders, which are relaxed. Keep your neck 'long' by looking down.

2 Keep looking down as you gently press your hips into the floor and pull your stomach in.

3 Gently, lift your head up (keep it independent of the body), focusing your eyes on the same point. Keep your feet on the floor.

4 Breathe in, and gently come down. Feel your buttocks contract slightly. Do not contract them too much, otherwise you're using your buttock muscles and not the stomach. Engaging the abdominals helps to strengthen your back and lift your body.

5 As you breathe out and lift, imagine that the crown of your head is going forward towards the wall in front of you. At the same time, let your hands 'float' off the ground. Do not lift your head towards the ceiling. Relax down again.

Watchpoints
• As you breathe out and lift, you should be able to get your fingers between your stomach and the floor.
• Whenever you do a back exercise, each time you breathe out your stomach goes into the spine (just as in the earlier abdominal exercises). If you lift too high and you feel your back shortening, you've gone too far.

ALTERNATE ARM AND LEG STRETCH FOR THE BACK

This exercise works your stomach and your back.

1 Lying on your stomach, imagine yourself in the shape of a rather small starfish. Your arms are slightly wider than your shoulders. Look down at the floor. Make sure your legs are comfortably apart and rotated slightly outwards. Don't force them though, simply lie there and just let your legs relax into their natural position.

2 Exhale and let your left leg and right arm gently float off the ground. Feel your stomach doing all the work.

3 Breathe in and lower.

4 Exhale as you change sides. Make sure that as your stomach goes in your tailbone drops. As you breathe, don't grip your bottom. Again, keep your legs straight and shoulders relaxed. Your arms and legs should be at the same height.

Repeat the exercise 10 times, alternating between sides.

Watchpoint
• Don't shorten your neck, grip your bottom, or lift your arm and leg too high off the ground. Don't think of 'lifting' – you should be 'lengthening' your arm and leg. The idea here is to do a diagonal stretch that strengthens and mobilizes the big back muscle between the base of one shoulder blade and the top of the opposite buttock.

KNEELING ARM AND LEG STRETCH

This exercise helps to improve balance. If it feels too difficult at the onset, you can start by lifting one arm, or one leg only.

1 Adopt the same position as the cat stretch (page 46), spine neutral and stomach gently in. Imagine someone's hand on your stomach.

2 Breathe out, and let your right arm and left leg gently float away. Don't lift too high. To avoid this, position something like a kitchen roll across the base of your spine. If you lift too high, it will fall off. Keep your pelvis neutral to avoid tilting from side to side. Keep looking at the same point on the floor, so that you don't shorten your neck. Relax back into the starting position.

Repeat, alternating arms and legs for 10 repetitions.

THE SWAN – ADVANCED BACK EXERCISE

All the same rules apply as in the Alternate Arm and Leg Stretch (page 49).

1 Once again, imagine you are a small starfish, lying on your front, with your arms and legs comfortably apart.

2 As you breathe out, lift both arms and both legs to the same height. Keep looking down throughout, and pull your stomach into your spine until you feel your tailbone drop.

Watchpoints
• As your stomach goes in, your pelvis relaxes back; as you breathe, don't grip your bottom.
• Keep your legs straight.
• Keep your shoulders relaxed, stomach in, legs and arms straight. Your arms and legs should be at the same height.

RELAXATION POSITION – CHILD'S POSE

Do this at the end of the back exercise sequence.

1 Sit back down on your heels with your arms close to your sides.

2 Gently pull your head into your chest and curl yourself into a small 'ball' until your forehead touches the ground.

3 Hold for a few seconds.

LEG EXERCISES

It is possible to create bulk by exercising the legs if you do not do enough stretching. Everyone wants their leg muscles to be long, lean and lengthened as opposed to tight and bunched. There are certain parts of the legs, particularly the quadriceps muscles above the knees, that get bigger due to excessive use, while the inside thighs and the hamstrings are usually undertoned. Many people tend to have overdeveloped quads, weak inside thighs and tight, but not strong, hamstrings.

The following exercises will help to strengthen, tone and condition your legs and help to make them more shapely. Any of these exercises can be done with ankle weights, but don't use anything heavier than 1 kilo (2 pounds 4 ounces). You want to tone and lengthen muscles, not build them up.

Leg strengthening exercises

INSIDE THIGH LIFT

This exercise will help tone flabby inside thighs (see picture, opposite).

1 Lie on your side, either with your hand supporting your head, or with your arm completely flat. If you choose to keep your arm flat, it may feel more comfortable to put a towel between your arm and ear.

2 Place your top leg forward, in front of the body. If this feels awkward, place a pillow under your knee. Put your other hand in front of you. The underneath leg (the one that is working) needs to be slightly forward, with the foot gently flexed. Again, don't lock your knee, but pull up the muscles, so that your leg is straight. If your legs are not straight, you'll be working your ankle and your foot much more than your inside thigh.

3 Breathe out, lift your underneath leg and hold.

4 Slowly lower the leg as you inhale. Don't lift your leg too high. Think of your leg going 'away', not up – because you want to lengthen and strengthen your muscles, not have them contracted and tight. As you lift and breathe out, your stomach pulls in, just like in the earlier stomach exercises. The energy is through the heel, working your inside thigh.

Do 10 on each side.

Watchpoint
• It's important to remember that, in all the leg exercises, the instigator is your stomach. This means you should feel your abdominal muscles working. The same applies to all the upper body exercises.

INSIDE THIGH CIRCLES

1 Lie on your side in the same position as the Inside Thigh Lift (page 53), either with your hand supporting your head, or with your arm completely flat. Place your top leg forward, in front of your body. Put your other hand in front of you. The underneath leg (the one that is working) needs to be slightly forward, with your foot gently pointed.

2 Gently point your foot. Breathe out and lift your underneath leg.

3 Slowly circle the leg in each direction. As you circle the leg, don't think of going up and down. Think of going out and away, so that you're almost touching the floor, as if you're circling around a fifty pence piece.

Do 10 little circles each way on each leg.

Watchpoint
• The knee is gently pulled up, the leg is reaching away, and you're circling down and away, not up.

OUTER THIGH LIFT

This exercise works the outer thighs and buttocks.

1 Lie on your side in the same position as the Inside Thigh Lift
(page 53), either with your hand supporting your head, or with your
arm completely flat. Put your other hand in front of you. This time
your underneath leg is bent comfortably in front of you. The top leg is
straight, flexed and very slightly forward. If you've got any doubts
about your back arching, you can lean against a wall.

2 The top leg should start the exercise at hip height. Very gently
breathe out and lift the leg about 15 centimetres (6 inches). Don't turn
your toes towards the ceiling. Keep your foot facing forward, gently
flexed. When you breathe out and lift, focus on the outer thigh and the
back of the leg.

Do 10 on each side.

OUTER THIGHS AND BUTTOCKS

1 Start this exercise in the same position as the Outer Thigh Lift (page 55). Make sure your top heel is in line with your hip.

2 Very gently breathe out and bring your leg forward, so that it's in line with the other knee.

3 Breathe in, and lift.

4 Breathe out, and lower and take the leg back.

This is quite a demanding exercise, so start with five on each side, then gradually build up to ten.

Watchpoints
• As you breathe out, and pull your leg forward, don't swing it. Think of your leg as a 'resistance', so that it is the stomach that is bringing your leg forward, up, down and back, as you tone the back of the thigh. Keep it in line with the other knee. Your hip stays back, your stomach stays in.
• If you find you get cramp in your hip, this exercise might not be for you.

OUTER THIGHS AND BUTTOCKS 2

1 In the same position as the Outer Thigh Lift (page 55), bend both of your knees so that they are comfortably in front of you. Gently flex your feet.

2 Lift the top leg, as if you're opening a fan. Then very gently breathe out, and squeeze the top leg straight.

3 As you breathe in, make a small bend in the knee.

4 Breathe out and squeeze straight. Remember – the emphasis is not on the bend, but on the squeeze. If you do a big bend, you'll be working your calves, not your bottom.

Do 10 on each side.

Watchpoint
• If you get cramp, this indicates that your muscles are fatigued and it is best to stop.

The following four leg exercises are done lying on the stomach. They can all be done with 1-kilo (2 pound 4 ounce) ankle weights.

HAMSTRING TONER AND STRENGTHENER

1 Lie on your stomach, with your head comfortably relaxed on your hands. If you prefer, keep your arms at your sides. Do whichever feels more comfortable. Keep your shoulders relaxed.

2 Very gently 'grip' your bottom. As you do so, you should feel your stomach going in and your tailbone drop.

3 Inhaling, bend your right leg and flex your foot.

4 Gently exhale and straighten, keeping the buttocks squeezed at all times.

Repeat 10 times then change legs. (The bend on this exercise is not important, it's just a preparation.)

BOTTOM TONER

1 Assume the same position on your stomach as in the Hamstring Toner and Strengthener exercise (above). In other words, lie on your stomach, with your head comfortably relaxed on your hands, or keep your arms at your sides.

2 With a straight leg, hip down, stomach in, keeping foot relaxed, with your buttocks gripped, very gently breathe out and lift your leg up. Then slowly bring it down. This works the buttock muscles, which are just under the cheek.

Do 10 repetitions on each leg.

BOTTOM TONER 2

1 Lie on your stomach, with your head comfortably relaxed on your hands, or keep your arms at your sides.

2 With a straight leg, hip down and stomach in, but this time keeping your foot softly flexed, with your buttocks gripped, very gently breathe out and lift your leg up. Then slowly bring it down.

Repeat 10 times on one leg and then the other.

BOTTOM TONER 3

This is the last exercise in this sequence. All the same rules apply as before.

1 Lie on your stomach, with your head comfortably relaxed on your hands, or keep your arms at your sides.

2 With a straight leg, hip down and stomach in, this time bend your leg and flex your foot as you lift, breathing out very gently. Then squeeze your leg to the ceiling and lower.

Repeat 10 times on one leg and then the other.

Watchpoints
- At no point in any of the last three exercises should your hip-bones leave the mat.
- If you feel your back arch, place a rolled towel beneath your stomach.

Leg stretches

It is vital that you do leg stretches after you've done any leg strengthening work. They are especially important if you have any back problems. If you've got a tight back, you may have tight legs. Sometimes it's difficult to know which comes first – a bad back and tight hamstrings, or tight hamstrings resulting in a bad back. Also, if you do have back problems you are likely to have a pelvic imbalance, which is often caused by overtight gluteal muscles, hip flexors and quadriceps, so that your pelvis is not in line. If you can get your body in line, you'll feel much more comfortable, and you will avoid a lot of problems.

Hold all stretches for 30 seconds.

BACK AND HIP – GLUTEAL STRETCH

1 Lie down on your back. If it feels more comfortable, place a towel under your head.

2 Cross your knees and hold onto your ankles.

3 Very gently pull your heels into your bottom. Do this for 30 seconds with the right leg on top, then 30 seconds with the left leg on top.

Repeat four times in total.

Watchpoints
- Don't let your bottom lift – it should stay 'weighted' to the ground.
- Don't hold onto your feet – hold onto your ankles.

BACK AND HIP – GLUTEAL STRETCH 2

This is a slightly more advanced version of the previous gluteal stretch exercise (page 60). It will help to release the hips.

1 Lying on your back with your legs bent (feet in the air), very gently cross the right ankle over the left knee (feet in the air). Make sure it's the ankle, and not the toes.

2 Gently, keeping your knee open, bend the left leg into the chest and feel a stretch on the right leg. Remember, on all the stretches, you should only feel a stretch on the working leg.

3 Hold for 30 seconds, change legs and repeat four times.

Watchpoint
• With both the gluteal stretch exercises, if you feel a strain in your back – stop. This means that you're working your legs too hard.

QUADRICEPS STRETCH (ADVANCED)

This exercise will stretch the quadricep muscles at the front of your thighs. Hold all stretches for 30 seconds.

1 Kneel down on your right leg. Extend the left leg in front with the knee bent and directly over the ankle.

2 Clasp your back foot with both hands, bend your knee and pull the foot towards your bottom. Keep your stomach in and don't arch your back.

3 Hold for 30 seconds.

Repeat four times, alternating legs.

LYING CALF STRETCH

1 Lie on your back, then bend your knees into your chest.

2 Place your hand behind the calf of the leg that you're working, and stretch the leg towards the ceiling. Keep your foot flexed.

3 Hold for 30 seconds.

Repeat four times, alternating legs.

STANDING CALF STRETCH

1 Stand up straight.

2 Take a step forward with your right leg, bend the knee slightly, and feel the stretch down through the back leg. Keep your heel down on the back leg. Do not bounce.

3 Hold for 30 seconds.

Repeat four times, alternating legs.

STANDING HAMSTRING STRETCH

1 Place your foot (gently flexed) on a chair and extend your leg. Keep the standing leg slightly bent and your stomach in. Neck and shoulders are relaxed. Hips are level.

2 Slide your hands down towards your foot. You should feel the stretch in the muscle between the knee and the hip.

3 Hold for 30 seconds.

Repeat four times, alternating legs.

LYING HAMSTRING STRETCH

For this exercise, most people need to place a towel beneath the head.

1 Lie on a mat or towel.

2 Start with both feet on the floor, knees bent, making sure you have equal weight down through both feet. The arms are beside you and the pelvis is in the neutral position.

3 Very gently bend your right knee into the chest. Grasp the back of your thigh with your left hand.

4 Grasp the back of your calf with your right hand and gently unfold, straightening that leg with a flexed foot, and ease the leg towards you. You'll know if you are doing it wrong if your bottom lifts. If this is impossible, instead of using your hands take a towel, place it around your calf and ease the leg towards you, keeping your neck and shoulders relaxed.

Do the right, then the left leg, and repeat, a minimum of twice on each side, holding for 30 seconds.

Watchpoint
• Don't pull on your leg so that your bottom leaves the floor, because your pelvis will twist. You want to flex the foot without overly tensing the feet, and gently straighten that knee. It is more important to get the knee straighter than to bring the leg closer to you.

INNER THIGH STRETCH

If you find this exercise difficult, sit on a cushion at first.

1 Sit on the floor with the soles of your feet together and your stomach in. Hold onto both ankles.

2 Gently drop your chin to your chest, relax your shoulders and let your knees drop to the sides.

3 Hold for 30 seconds.

Repeat four times.

ADVANCED INNER THIGH STRETCH

1 Lie on your back, with your legs up a wall.

2 Let your legs fan out to the sides as far as is comfortable. Make sure your stomach is in, and your tailbone dropped. If you feel any pain in your knees, stop.

3 Hold for 30 seconds. Bring your legs back together.

Repeat four times.

HIP FLEXOR AND FRONT OF THE THIGH EXERCISE

This exercise stretches the front of your thigh and the quadriceps muscle.

1 Kneeling in a lunge position, holding on to a chair to stabilize your weight, have one foot in front of you with the knee bent. The knee should be directly above the ankle. If the foot is behind the knee, you may strain your knee. You can either have the toes pointing directly forward or at '10 to 2' (think of your foot as a clock hand.) Do whatever feels more comfortable for you. Due to the way in which your lower leg is aligned, the position of comfort may vary.

2 Kneeling on the other leg, with the foot behind you, very gently pull your stomach in. Press your hips forward and feel a stretch down the front of the thigh. At no point arch your back. Your stomach is pulled in, your shoulders are relaxed – imagine that someone has one hand on your stomach gently pushing your stomach in and the other hand on your bottom, which is being gently pushed forward to stabilize your spine.

Repeat the exercise twice on each side, alternating legs.

Note
If you find this exercise comfortable, you can go on to take your hands away from the chair, put them on your knee and take slightly more of a lean back to get a stronger stretch, but not at the expense of arching your back, straining your knee or letting your stomach protrude.

Watchpoint
• Don't kneel on a hard floor because you may hurt your knee. With exercises involving the knees, if you have any knee pain at any time, stop. Pain in the knee is not a good sign in any exercise.

UPPER BODY

In my experience as a Pilates teacher, all women want a beautiful upper back, gorgeous shoulders, lovely arms and triceps. The following exercises will tone your back, arms, shoulders and chest.

The spine is the central structure of the body. Tight or weak back muscles will eventually lead to problems. Taking steps to strengthen one's back is insurance for the future. A strong back and centre go hand in hand to present an upright and confident person.

You can do second sets when your body builds up to it and follow them with the stretches, which are absolutely essential after performing upper body work. Proper stretching will prevent you from having rounded shoulders and tight muscles.

One combination could be press-ups, dips and then repeat. An alternative would be a bicep curl, tricep press and then repeat.

PRESS-UPS

This exercise is a slight variation of a press-up, which I use a lot in my studio.

1 On your hands and knees, make a square with the body. Do not kneel on a hard surface – use a towel or an exercise mat. Your knees should be under the hips, and the hands under the shoulders. Cross one hand over the other. Check that the neck is in line, and that the back is not arched. Pull the stomach in. Do not lock the elbows.

2 Very gently, using the entire body, tip yourself slightly forward over the arms. Do not arch your back. It is very natural, when assuming the press-up position, to allow your head to drop. However, try to keep the head in a neutral position, neither forward nor backward.

3 Do six repetitions with the right hand on top, then the left. Work up to 10 or 12 with each hand on top. Very gently breathe in as you bend the arms, bringing the chest down. Breathe out as you push away.

Note
If possible, do the press-ups in front of a mirror. When you press down, your head should not lower and your chin should not stick out. When you start, you will feel your weight rocking slightly forwards and backwards. Try to stabilize the weight over the arms so that you get the most strengthening through the upper back, the shoulders, the triceps and biceps muscles in the arms.

DIPS

1 Using a chair placed against a wall for support, stand with your back towards the chair.

2 Bend your knees and rest the heels of your palms on the seat of the chair behind you. Have your hands wide enough apart so that your shoulders don't feel pinched together. Fingers should be facing forward. Your knees should be over your ankles. If they're not, you'll be using your thighs as opposed to the backs of your arms.

3 As you breathe in, bend your arms; as you breathe out, straighten your arms. Make sure as you do the dips that you're sliding your bottom down the edge of the chair and that you're not sliding forward, as the body will automatically prefer to do, and taking the strain in the front of the thighs.

You might only be able to start with eight repetitions; gently build up to 25.

BICEPS CURL

1 Adopt a standing position. Holding a 2-kilo (4 pound 8 ounce) weight in each hand, breathe in and then bend one arm up to shoulder level.

2 Breathe out and straighten your arm to waist level. Try not to rock as you do this.

Repeat 10 to 15 times with alternate arms.

TRICEPS PRESS

1 Face a firm chair and make a square with your body by placing your left hand and knee on the chair, keeping your right leg straight on the ground. Keep your neck in line with the rest of your body.

2 Holding a hand weight in your right arm, lift it up as high as you can behind you, keeping the elbow bent at a right angle, without twisting the body. Exhale as you straighten the arm behind you. Pause.

3 Bend your arm back again.

Repeat 10 to 15 times on each arm. You may do a second set.

LAT EXERCISE

Do not use your shoulders to do the work in this exercise.

1 Assume the same position as in the Triceps Press (page 71). In other words, face a firm chair and make a square with your body. Place your left hand and knee on the chair, keeping your right leg straight on the ground. Keep your neck in line with the rest of your body. All the same rules apply.

2 This time you're using your arm to pull up and down. As you 'pull', feel your lats doing all the work – imagine you're pulling up weeds.

Repeat 10 to 15 times on each arm. You may do a second set.

SHOULDER STRETCH

This stretch can be done seated or standing.

1 Cross one arm over the other, bring your palms towards you and clasp your hands together.

2 Gently push your elbows to the ceiling and feel your shoulders stretching. As you press your arms up, try to keep your shoulders down. Keep your elbows in line with your shoulders.

3 Hold for 10 seconds and then relax.

Repeat four times, alternating arms.

Watchpoint
• If you feel any cramp or discomfort in your shoulders or arms, you are not yet flexible enough to do this.

Arm exercises

The following arm exercises are done lying on your back. You should do them after your upper body work. They will help you to keep your shoulders flexible. Place a towel under your head if it feels more comfortable.

In all of these exercises remember to keep your back in a neutral position: don't let your ribs lift. Keep your feet hip-width apart, knees bent, with no tension in the lower back.

ARMS OPENING

1 Lie on your back and raise your arms above your chest. Your knees should be bent, with your feet flat on the floor.

2 Imagine you're a tulip, and as you breathe out, your arms gently open.

3 As you breathe in, bring your arms back together. Keep the curve in the elbows. Repeat 10 times, opening and closing.

BACKSTROKE

1 Lie on your back. Your knees should be bent, with your feet flat on the floor. Hold your arms over your chest. The palms face the wall in front of you. Keep your shoulders relaxed.

2 As you breathe out, simultaneously one arm goes down in front of you and one behind you.

3 Breathe in as you reverse the arms. Imagine you're doing the backstroke.

Repeat 20 times, 10 on each side.

ARM CIRCLES

1 Lie on your back and raise your arms above your chest. Your knees should be bent, with your feet flat on the floor.

2 With your arms stretched up above you, breathe out and make a circle with your arms, so that your hands touch the floor all the way behind you.

3 Bring your arms back and stretch towards your hips.

Repeat 10 circles one way and 10 going the other.

SHOULDER STRETCH

1 Lie on your back. Your knees should be bent, with your feet flat on the floor. Keep your shoulders relaxed.

2 Place one hand gently over the other, so that you're making a diamond shape with your elbows.

3 As you breathe out, take your arms as far back to the floor, past your ears, as you can without your back lifting.

Repeat 10 times, alternating the hand on top.

ROLLING UP AND DOWN THE WALL

This is a great way to relax at the end of any programme, but if you have any back pain don't do it.

1 Stand and lean your back against a wall. Remember always to keep the knees bent, otherwise you risk straining your back.

2 Breathe out, and very slowly drop your chin to your chest. It helps if you count as you do this. Start to roll your back down, as gently as you can. By the time you get to a count of eight, your shoulders should roll off the wall. If your legs start to shake, bend your knees a bit more. Roll down as far as you feel comfortable and count for 10–20 seconds. Your arms should now be hanging loosely by your sides like a puppet's.

3 Gently move your head from side to side.

4 Pause, and try to roll up, very slowly.

Repeat four times (twice down, twice up).

Watchpoint
• If you've got low blood pressure don't do this, or you might feel faint.

QUICK PROGRAMMES
FOR A BUSY DAY

Lifestyles can create polarization. In other words, we may go from 'living' at the gym to a total abstinence from any form of exercise, the most common reason being lack of time. I have tried to address this problem by weaving the following exercises into a busy day, making it easier to implement movement during your free time.

I have divided the exercises into three programmes: the Morning Energizer, Postural Awareness at Work, and Midday Break. There is a series of cards for each of these programmes, so you can have them handy whenever you are ready to do the exercises.

PROGRAMME 1:
MORNING ENERGIZER

Sleep is supposed to restore us; it is the time when the body regenerates itself. Despite its obviously therapeutic uses, some people don't sleep terribly well. They may have disturbed slumber or they may lie in bed in uncomfortable positions.

Often people wake up feeling lethargic, tight and tense. The six exercises in this programme focus on limbering and release, and will enable you to start your day in a positive frame of mind. Doing these gentle mobilizing exercises early in the day will reconstruct some of the body's internal alignment. They will wake you up, stimulate you and get your joints moving. They will also initiate the feeling of alignment – of standing up straight, feeling balanced and positive. All the exercises in this programme are done approximately 10 times.

Exercise mat or towel

In all the exercises that involve lying on the floor, it is recommended that you use an exercise mat, but a large bath towel will do. Don't do these exercises on a wooden floor with only a towel. A bath towel placed on a carpet, however, should give enough support to your spine.

Concentrating on limbering and release, this 10-minute programme of morning stretches focuses on releasing the lower spine and hips and gently loosening the upper body. The spine, the upper and lower back, and the muscles in the backs of your legs will be released. One movement, based on a classic Pilates exercise, opens up your spine and releases through your discs. Hip rotations will lubricate your hips. The arm exercises will open your shoulder girdle and start getting you to focus on breathing. Finally, there is a side stretch done with a towel to stretch and open up generally. The Morning Energizer should make you feel physical liberation and a spiritual awakening.

ROLLING UP LIKE A BALL

This exercise can be difficult; work your way into it. Many people don't have a lot of flexibility in the spine, so you might have a problem in getting back up again. If this is the case, come back up normally and start the roll again. Rolling up like a ball is the exercise I do first when I exercise.

1 Sit holding onto your shins, with your knees bent.

2 Curl up like a ball. As you breathe out, roll backwards.

3 As you breathe in, roll up to a seated position.

Repeat the whole exercise 10 times.

Watchpoint
• Try to keep the heels close to your bottom all the way through, and relax your shoulders. As you breathe out and roll back, the stomach pulls in. Do not roll too high up on the neck.

HIP MOBILITY EXERCISE

As we get older the hips get tighter, and there is less articulation in the hip socket.

1 Lie on a large towel or an exercise mat. Keep the feet together and hold on just below the knees. If you feel uncomfortable, put a towel behind your head. The body should not move, the head is resting.

2 Holding on below the knees, keeping the toes together, rotate your hips 10 times in one direction and 10 times in the other, to lubricate your hips.

3 Keeping the toes together, start with the knees apart. As you breathe normally, they come into the chest, then they open and come around. It doesn't matter in which direction you go. This exercise will also help to warm your lumbar spine and the entire pelvis area. You may feel a gentle stretch in your inside thighs if they're tight. Don't force this feeling of stretch. Just feel the mobilization. You're getting blood to flow through your hips and releasing tension through your pelvis. Don't have your legs too far away from you. Keep your knees over your hips. Your legs do not hang off your body. Your tailbone is heavy and supported by the mat or towel at all times.

Watchpoint
- Hold onto your shins and thighs, never the knees.

FULL BODY WAKE-UP STRETCH

You'll feel this stretch in the back of your legs, your hamstrings, calf muscles, feet and shoulders. You may feel a stomach stretch as well.

1 Lie on your back with a towel behind your head and flex your feet – your toes pointing up towards your knees. Hold your hands, with your fingers entwined.

2 As you breathe in, the elbows bend so the hands almost touch the crown of the head.

3 As you breathe out, stretch your arms as far away from you as you can, flex your feet and stretch.

4 Breathe in, bend your elbows, relax, breathe out and stretch.

Do approximately 10 repetitions.

Note

You can either do this exercise with the hands crossed or the fingers interlaced. Breathe in, breathe out and stretch. As you breathe out and stretch, the shoulders shrug up towards the ears. As you breathe in, relax the shoulders and let them drop. The hands come towards the crown of your head or forehead, and the legs relax. As you breathe out, the fingers and hands stretch away, the shoulders lift and the flexed feet stretch towards the other end of the room. The body is stretched and energized.

Warm-ups for the shoulders and back

The following two exercises in the programme are about postural awareness. At this point do not stand on a towel unless you feel very secure. This exercise is better done with bare feet, so that you can feel the contact with the floor. This exercise is about coordination, where both arms work rhythmically, alternating.

SHOULDERS AND BACK 1

1 Stand with your feet hip-width apart. Relax your feet. Make sure the weight is evenly placed over your feet and try not to sink either forwards or backwards. The toes should be relaxed and lengthened as if they're softening into sand. When you're standing upright the stomach is gently pulled in, the tailbone drops and the pelvis is in neutral.

2 Start with the arms naturally relaxed at your sides. They don't hang behind you, they gently soften, as if your middle finger is stretching down the outside of your thigh, lengthening away. In this position your hands are just in front of you. Your shoulders are relaxed and your head is in a neutral position. Don't let your head drop forward or back. Let it sit on top of your shoulders. Use visualization techniques and think of your head as a blossom sitting on the stem of a plant. The head is just softly there. Your knees are released.

3 As you breathe out, one arm reaches to the ceiling, and the other arm gently reaches to the wall behind you without any shift in the feet, the pelvis, the upper back or the neck. If you're feeling that shift, you are taking the movement too far for your initial flexibility.

This exercise can be done either 10 times (5 on each side), or 20 (which is 10 on each side), alternating the arms.

SHOULDERS AND BACK 2

This exercise targets the same area as the previous exercise. It is about coordination: you want both arms to start and end at the same point. You don't want one arm to begin before the other.

1 Adopt the same starting position as in Shoulders and Back 1 (page 82). Start with the same postural alignment, no gripping of the feet, no tensing of the buttocks – everything is relaxed and calm. Straighten both your arms and bring them in front of you with the tips of the little fingers touching.

2 As you breathe out, take a slice and reach to the corners of the room. The arms stay straight all the way through. Breathe in, breathe out, then slice, reaching for the corners of the room.

Note
After you've done this exercise 10 times, you may do a few on the diagonal. You slice, gently twist and the head follows. You will feel a gentle stretch across the chest and some stretching through the shoulders.

Watchpoint
• With any of the arm exercises, at no point should you lock your elbows. The joints are in line: the shoulders, the elbows, the wrists, all the fingers – don't break at the wrist.

WAIST STRETCH

1 Stand in the same position as in the Shoulders and Back 1 exercise (page 82), with your feet hip-width apart. Hold a folded hand-towel nice and wide between your shoulders.

2 Breathe out and stretch to one side.

3 Breathe in, straighten up, and breathe out to stretch to the other side. Don't lift your shoulders up to your ears, and stretch only as far as you don't shorten on the underneath side.

Do about 10 repetitions on each side.

Watchpoints
• Your weight should be evenly balanced over both feet. You'll know you've gone too far if you feel one foot coming off the floor. The weight is over the second toe, as in all of the standing exercises. The hips don't move very much because it is a waist-energizing stretch. Breathe out as you take the stretch, breathe into the centre and breathe out as you change.
• The waist stretch is related to core strength. You engage your abdominals to stabilize your pelvis and your spine during a gentle waist stretch; the body does not collapse from side to side. Keep the weight evenly distributed over both feet for the duration of the exercise and don't allow yourself to tip from one side to the other.

PROGRAMME 2: POSTURAL AWARENESS AT WORK

With the exercises in this programme you will maximize posture and energy levels in environmentally unfriendly conditions. You will learn to sit and stand correctly throughout the day. New habits will form and, once learned, will be hard to break. Your body will feel comfortable and well-balanced, freeing you to be mentally alert.

Generally people sit badly. They sink into their hips when they sit down. Most people are not as active as they should be because of the restrictions in their daily lives. These exercises will take you back to basics, recreating the way you sit. The emphasis in these exercises is not on complicated movement but on visualization.

You should be sitting at your desk, with your chair at the right level, with your feet grounded through the floor, and equal pressure down through both feet. Your lower back is supported in the chair, the upper back floating above with no tension. A shoulder stretch has also been included in this programme, which will release tense shoulders. You then breathe into your stomach and, on the exhalation, you contract your stomach into the back of the chair, concentrating on feeling that movement of internal support as you grow taller and more confident.

SITTING PROPERLY AND BREATHING CORRECTLY

1 Sit with your back supported by a chair. Your tailbone is heavy and both feet are evenly placed on the floor.

2 Feel that you are in contact from your centre directly down through your feet into the floor. You're going to channel your energies from your centre out through the crown of your head. Ensure that your shoulders are relaxed; your arms are relaxed because your middle back is supported. Your tailbone will drop and your abdominals will naturally pull back towards your spine.

3 Try to think of your head sitting naturally on top of your shoulders, not pushing forward and not pushing back.

4 Now practise your breathing. Place your fingers on your lower abdominals, the space between your pubic bone and your navel. As you breathe in the stomach gently expands, filling with oxygen. As you breathe out the stomach pulls away from your fingers and settles back into the chair, your navel pulls away from your fingers and you feel the energy going in to support the lower back.

Repeat the breathing exercise 10 times.

Watchpoint
• If you force your shoulders back and your lower back arches away from the chair, you will know that your shoulders are still too rounded for you to be able to maintain this position and be anatomically correct.

FOOT LIFTS

1 Sit in a chair, as in the Sitting Properly and Breathing Correctly exercise (page 86). You can either have your fingers on your abdomen in the same place as before or allow your arms to hang naturally beside you.

2 As you breathe in your abdomen gently softens or expands into your fingers, and as you breathe out you very gently let one foot float off the floor, feeling the connection of the navel to the spine.

3 Place the foot down, make sure you have even pressure through both feet again, and change legs. The coordination is important. The start-off foot lifts very slowly; eventually you will be able to do the lifts faster so that the interchange emanates from a stable pelvis and a strong abdomen.

Note
Initially the change from one leg to the other might feel unstable if you don't have the core strength to coordinate alternate leg lifts automatically. The feet should float off the floor.

Do 10 lifts with each leg, alternating each time.

Watchpoint
• If you lift your feet too high, you will feel your pelvis sink back into the chair and you'll lose that postural alignment. Your tailbone will tuck underneath and your back will curl. For this exercise wear no shoes or flat shoes.

RELAX YOUR ANKLES

This exercise will relax your ankles, calves and feet, and it will give you a conscious feeling of the connection between your body and the earth.

1 Sit in a chair, as in the Sitting Properly and Breathing Correctly exercise (page 86). Slip your shoes off, cross one knee over the other and gently circle your ankle very slowly, so that you take six seconds to circle the ankle in one direction, approximately six to eight times.

2 Change directions and repeat, then do the same thing with the other ankle.

Watchpoint
• Try to keep your toes relaxed, don't grip with them. Do not move the bones in your lower leg (the tibia and fibula). Think of your ankle bones as pebbles that you're gently shaking. While you're circling the ankle, the pebbles are lubricating and relaxing. If you tense your foot and lower leg, this process will not happen. Your ankles and calves will feel warmer after this exercise, if it is completed slowly and rhythmically.

SHOULDER STRETCH 2

1 Sit in a chair, as in the Sitting Properly and Breathing Correctly exercise (page 86). All the same rules apply: stomach pulled in, tailbone dropped, both feet evenly balanced on the floor. Think of your energy evenly placed down through both feet.

2 Very gently, place your right hand on your left shoulder blade, palm facing down. Take your other hand behind and underneath and try to reach and connect your fingers behind you. If you can't do this initially, don't worry, aim to do it eventually.

3 Without arching your back or sticking your chest out, gently open out the right or the left top arm to stretch. Keep the neck long.

4 Do the other side, then five times on each side, alternating sides.

NECK STRETCH

This neck stretch should not be done more than four times.

1 Sit in your chair, with your feet comfortably apart. Gently place the palm of your right hand not on your neck, but behind the crown of your head.

2 Drop your chin towards your chest without leaning forward, look at your big toe and gently press your head against your hand; feel the neck stretching. Hold for 20 seconds.

3 Relax, do the stretch on the left and then once more on either side.

> **Watchpoint**
> • The middle back should be supported, tailbone dropped; don't let the chin go forward.

PROGRAMME 3:
MIDDAY BREAK

The human mind and body don't function at their best after working for eight consecutive hours. You need to have a space or a break in your working day, whether it's a brisk walk or reading a newspaper. A change of environment – physical or mental – will recharge your batteries. Your mind and body will be clearer and you'll feel less sluggish in your working environment.

An active aerobic break combined with stretches and body-releasing exercises makes a lunch break a good time to rejuvenate and recharge. 'Aerobic' is a very general term that can indicate anything from climbing the stairs to taking a short walk.

This programme is a restart and refocus. It involves a lot of stretching. It will address the areas that are tight from sitting and working, and will be especially helpful for those who work in front of a computer screen.

You will stand up and do some very simple foot exercises, such as grasping the floor with your toes and releasing, followed by calf stretches, a shoulder stretch and a cat stretch. There is also a stretch in which you stand in the doorway and release your shoulders. This focuses the energy away from areas of work-induced tightness so you can feel relaxed and liberated when you lunch. You can then enjoy your lunch break, because you will have rid yourself of work-related muscular stress.

DOMING

Doming is better done with bare feet.

1 Stand up on the floor. Very gently lift one foot so that it's just resting on the heel. As you place your foot on the ground, spread your toes and try to separate them. Ideally they will all spread and separate at the same time. (Imagine doing doming with your hand: you lift and separate your fingers as you place them down.)

2 Holding your toes down, draw up the arch underneath your foot. Relax.

3 As you flex onto the heel and spread the toes again, imagine having chewing gum under the ball of your foot. You draw your toes up – without gripping the floor – and relax. In the beginning you might get cramp in your foot.

Do 10 repetitions with each foot.

Watchpoint
• Do not let your toes become 'clawed' in this exercise.

CALF STRETCH

Again, this exercise is done without shoes.

1 Stand a little way back from your office desk or chair, with your feet hip-width apart. Without moving your feet, lean forward and put your hands on the desk or chair for support. Your shoulders should be down, your stomach in, and your tailbone dropped. Don't arch your back or stick out your ribs. Keep your shoulders down and your head 'floating' on top of your body.

2 Now do a very simple calf stretch by taking a step forward with one leg and feeling a stretch down the back of the other, the heel touching the floor. Hold for 30 seconds.

3 Do the other leg, then repeat the stretch on both legs again.

Watchpoint
• Remember that your stomach should be in and your tailbone should be dropped.

SHOULDER ROTATION

This exercise will open up your shoulders. It can be done seated in an office chair, but the preferred position is standing against a door frame or wall.

1 Stand up and lean with your knees bent and middle back against the wall.

2 Slide down, keeping the knees bent. Your weight should be placed evenly over the feet, which are not tense. Your middle back and the space between your shoulder blades should touch the wall for support. Do not push your head back or you will feel your middle back and shoulder blades come off the wall.

3 Breathing normally, gently place your hands on your shoulders. This exercise consists of four movements: circle arms forward, trying to get the elbows to touch, lift up towards the ears, circle as far back as you can without any of your middle back coming off the wall. When you have completed the movement, you then circle the other way. Back, up, around and down.

Do 10 repetitions in each direction.

Watchpoint
• Keep your middle back and the space between the shoulder blades on the wall.

HAND EXERCISE

This exercise will help those people with stiff hands or people suffering from Repetitive Strain Injury (RSI). However, if you are suffering from RSI or any other injury, check with your doctor before beginning these exercises.

1 Sit or stand with your shoulders relaxed.

2 Stretch your hands very gently and bring each finger to the thumb, beginning with the little finger. Stretch each of your fingers as much as you can.

Note
You can either do this exercise with your hands in front of you or behind you. The movement is exactly the same, but at the same time you circle the wrist. Think of Balinese dancers. This exercise also works on coordination.

Watchpoint
- Keep the shoulders and elbows relaxed.

CAT STRETCH AT THE DESK

Using an office desk or chair, this exercise will release your lower back and stretch out your shoulders. Shoes should be off unless you're in flat shoes. Do not do this exercise in heels.

1 Stand as far away from your desk or chair as you can while still resting your palms on it.

2 Bend your knees slightly and keep them bent. Weight goes down evenly through both feet.

3 Breathe out, curl your chin into your chest, your stomach into your spine. Stretch out your lower back. This will counteract the effects of being seated for long periods of time, and get the blood flowing as you open your spine.

4 As you breathe in, press your chest down; your bottom goes up and the head gently lengthens back.

Watchpoint
• If you feel the neck crunching or your vocal cords contracting, you've taken your head too far back. There should be no discomfort in your neck.

SHOULDER STRETCH 3

1 Again, stand as far away from your desk or chair as you can with your palms resting on it.

2 Bend your knees slightly and keep them bent. Weight goes down evenly through both feet.

3 For this shoulder stretch, keep the ears between the arms. Holding onto the desk or chair, press your chest down and stretch your arms to give your shoulders, neck and upper arms a good stretch. Don't worry if you feel a little ache in your upper arms, because it is 'referred pain' from stretching out your upper back.

Watchpoint
• Keep your knees bent and your head between your arms.